Legal & Disclaimer

Journey Out of Depression

Inspiring Story of One Woman's Journey to Overpower Depression and Anxiety, The Drug Free Way

Foreword

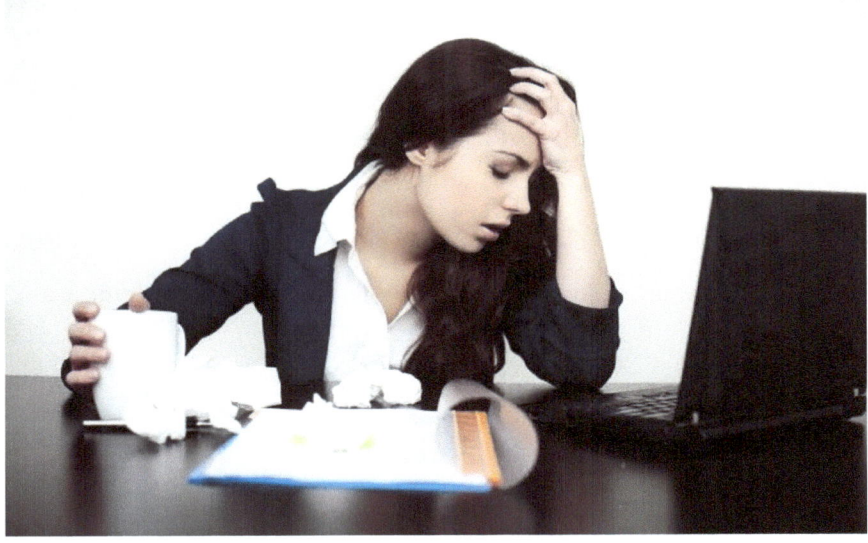

If left unchecked, depression and anxiety can overwhelm you. We must fight back and overpower them, and subdue them, so that they do not come back to haunt our life. In my previous book "***Overpowering Depression and Anxiety - The Drug-Free and Sustainable Way***", I outlined a 5-pillar strategy to prepare readers to fight depression and anxiety in a manner that is drug free, as well as sustainable so that it does not come back to haunt our life.

This book is written to complement it. When I was writing that book, it contains a lot of theories and concepts, but like all other non-fiction books, can be a little dry and filled with theories that many people may just dismiss it as "another one of those many books out there that talks about similar thing".

I really want people to benefit from that book, and I have been thinking about how I can make it more compelling for people to read and remember well the pillars and concepts that I shared there. After a while, I realize that the best way may be to tell a story that is based on the key concepts which I share in this book, and make the story as interesting and compelling as possible. People remember stories much better than facts. So if the story is compelling, and people remembers it better, then hopefully they can better utilize the steps that I outlined in the other book, and I would have fully achieved my objectives.

Thus I hope you will enjoy the story about that I am going to share with you in this book. It is about how a woman suffering from depression actually walk out of depression using the 5 pillar methods that I shared in the other book. And you get the most from the story as well as the concept if you read this book along with the other book. It does not matter which sequence you read, though the more logical sequence is to read the theory first, then read the story and see how it was applied.

I hope you will enjoy, and also benefit from this book.... Happy Reading.

Chapter 1 – "I Don't Feel So Good...."

Foggy with sleep, she tried to make sense of the incessant buzz that was echoing in her head. It was a familiar buzz that she knew she had heard before; shrill and irritating like a muffled power drill. She willed it to stop – and it did. Laura opened her eyes to see her husband Alex reach over her to turn off the alarm clock that was on her side of the bed. Was it morning already? She had gone to bed early last night and had immediately fallen into a heavy, dreamless sleep. But she was still tired. In fact, she couldn't move. Her whole body felt heavy and lifeless. Rather than waking up refreshed and energized after her early night, she felt worse.

The bedclothes rustled as Alex sat up in bed. Seeing her awake, he ruffled her hair, kissed her lightly and jumped out of bed. Stretching and yawning loudly, he walked into the bathroom and immediately after she heard the shower running.

Usually, she would go down to the kitchen to put the coffee on and lay our breakfast, then go back up to shower and dress for work. Instead, she lay there, staring up at the ceiling. Lately, she had been finding it harder and harder to get up in the morning. She felt safe in her little cocoon of bed clothes. Oh, what luxury to be able to stay in in the warm bed, sleep throughout the day and just forget about life.

This was strange because she had always been a morning person; cheerful, energetic, full of vigor and health. Until recently, she had loved her job as a top sales coordinator at a busy property company. She loved the fast-paced, sometimes frantic workdays, the challenge of meeting and even exceeding her weekly target and she had never minded the long hours or the pressure, until these past few weeks when she had started having these weird feelings and thoughts. She would be typing something on her computer or speaking with a customer on the phone when suddenly she would feel a rush of deep sadness, like there was a big empty hole inside her, a deep sense of loss that was beyond tears. At other times she would feel a bone-crushing weariness where she longed to put her head down on her desk and just sleep. More and more often she would find herself wondering, what's the purpose of this mindless, meaningless struggle we call life? What are we all rushing madly to achieve? Aren't we all going to die in the end?

The feelings of loss and despair were especially heightened when she and Alex watched the evening news. War, suicide bombings, floods, earthquakes, shootings, murder, rape…chaos death and destruction everywhere. Alex would shake his head in bewilderment. "Madness", he would mutter. The world has gone totally utterly mad!" But to Laura, the images on the TV screen were like a message specifically for her, enforcing her thoughts that yes, life was all pointless.

The sudden silence interrupted her thoughts. The shower had stopped. Alex would be out and expecting his coffee. She took a deep breath, threw back the bed covers and literally hauled herself out of bed. Every muscle, every bone, every cell in her body felt drained and lifeless. Should she be worried? Should she see a doctor? Should she tell Alex? No, no, why make a fuss? She's been pushing herself pretty hard at work lately, filling in for Jenny who was on maternity leave. All she needed was a nice weekend of rest and relaxation.

As a matter of fact, now that she was up and out of bed, she was feeling better already. It was easy to go downstairs, put on the coffee and set out cereal, bowls and milk. The daily routine had started.

Back upstairs, she showered quickly and for some reason did not feel like taking her usual time over her hair and makeup. Standing before the closet door the feeling hit her again, a wave of listlessness and emptiness that left her standing there staring into the closet, unable to make a simple decision: what to wear. That was another thing she had noticed lately; he inability to focus and make quick decisions. What was the point, anyway? What did it matter? She was going to go sit at a desk for eight hours selling houses over the phone… "Honey, we're running late!" Alex had been driving her to work on his way to the office to save on gas and he liked to leave early to avoid the rush hour. Not knowing or caring what she grabbed from the closet, she dressed quickly and ran downstairs.

Sitting next to Alex in the car, Laura pretended to listen to his casual conversation - but she was having a mental conversation of her own. The closet episode had really shaken her. "You're not stupid," she was saying to herself. "In fact, you're pretty smart. You have a college degree; you read a lot, keep up with current affairs and have a high-level job. Everybody's always telling you how intelligent you are. You know what's wrong with you. You're displaying the classic symptoms of depression. Stop telling yourself that this is a mild case of the blues. The symptoms are getting worse. You're in denial…"

At that precise moment, Alex reached out and stroked her face. "Why so glum?" he asked in his familiar, mildly sarcastic tone. "You're always quire happy and chirpy setting off for another day in the rat race."

She took his hand in hers and pressed it hard, "Alex, I think I need to see a doctor…:

Chapter 2 – Meeting an Old Friend

Warm sunlight warmed the autumn chill in the air as Laura strolled around the downtown streets, shopping bags in her hand. It was Alex's birthday and they were having a small dinner party for a few close friends. She had finished her shopping but continued walking, stopping occasionally to look absent-mindedly into a shop window. She hoped Alex would like his birthday gifts: a new shirt in his favorite blue color, a book on his latest passion Ancient Egypt and a new carrier bag for his laptop. Should she buy a card as well? There was a gift shop nearby that sold romantic cards…She knew she was stalling. She had to get home to get everything ready but she had one more place to go – the drugstore, to refill her medication prescription.

Three weeks had passed since her confession to Alex that she needed help. And he had been absolutely wonderful, a real rock during these past weeks. He had immediately booked an appointment with a top psychiatrist and took the day off to go with he. He apologized over and over for not noticing what she was going through. The big new project at work had been taking up all his thoughts. His accompanying her to the doctor made up for that. She had been dreading having to go alone.

The doctor was nice enough although a little detached. He asked her to describe what she was felling and typed notes on his laptop. He confirmed that she was suffering from depression.

Thankfully, her condition had not yet become chronic but the recurring cycles were a sign that the problem could be serious if not checked. He said the medication was the best option for her case, and proceeded to prescribed several. He assured her that the drugs were the quickest and most common method to deal with her type of depression, and that any other doctor would prescribe the same ones. He would start decreasing the dosage in a couple of months once there were signs of improvement.

And there had been improvement. She was sleeping better most night, her energy levels were higher and her bouts of indecision were completely gone. She still felt fatigued and listless some days but not the crippling weariness she had felt before. And despite her improved mood, she still felt that strange emptiness inside her. She laughed and smiled less often and her natural optimism and zest for life were not what they once were. Sometimes she felt sadness so deep that it was beyond tears. Still, she was grateful for the improvement and hopeful that she would soon be her old self again.

"Give yourself time." Alex had said. "It's a long process and you're so much better already. Take it slow and just know I'm with you every step of the way." Dear, beloved Alex! Yes, he was right. It would take perseverance, patience, and the medications needed time to work.

The medications…she hated picking them up. They were a reminder that something was wrong with her, that the journey was going to be long and slow. More importantly, they reminded her of the emptiness and loneliness that would not go away.

But she knew she had to be getting home soon so she turned back and walked to the drugstore. She handed her prescription to the clerk. Another reason she hated coming to the drugstore was that it reminded her of the strain the medications were putting on their finances. The stuff was not cheap, and the costs had run into more than they could really afford. Alex reassured her that he was making more than enough to cover the expense but she worried nonetheless. This was money they should be putting away towards the future, towards starting a family and buying a bigger house. Alex refused to let her pay a penny out of her own salary. "I'm the head of the house and I pay for everything needed under my roof."

She was standing at the counter lost in her thoughts when suddenly she heard a voice saying her name. She turned to see a tall, beautiful woman smiling at her. She stared at the woman's face which seemed familiar, but she couldn't quite place it. The woman had tanned, glowing skin, light hazel eyes and sun-streaked reddish blond hair pulled back into a long ponytail.

The woman chuckled "I don't wear as much makeup as I used to in high school but come on; I recognized you right away!" The deep, bubbly voice was familiar and looking closer, Laura recognized her old high school classmate, Serene.

They had been best friends and had hung out together a lot, walking to school, sitting together in class, going out with other friends. They had lost touch soon after graduation when Serene's family had moved to another state.

"Oh my gosh, Serene!" she exclaimed; "Of all the people I least expected to run into!" They stood chatting for a while and Serne suggested they have a quick cup of coffee at the next door coffee shop. At that moment, the clerk handed Laura her prescription and she saw Serene looking at the medications. "Oh, you're taking drugs for depression are you?" She had always been blunt in an open and honest kind of way with no intention of being offensive or mean and Laura noted that she hadn't changed. Laura nodded putting the medication in her purse. "My doctor says it's the complaint of our modern times. It's almost as common as the common cold. I hope I won't be on them for too long." Serene looked at her for a long moment. "I hope so too." she said.

Over coffee, they quickly filled each other in on what they had been up to. Serene had moved back to town where her husband of two years was starting a small law firm. They had both decided it was the best place to settle down and start a family. Laura spoke about her marriage to Alex five years ago following a one-year romance, his job as a software developer and her own job.

As they chatted, Laura found herself wondering at how much Serene had changed. She had always been pretty but now she was perfectly stunning. Even without makeup and with her hair pulled back, she radiated an almost unearthly, radiant beauty. She was dressed simply but elegantly and appeared poised and confident. Laura became aware of her own hair that needed washing, her ragged nails and the old sweatshirt and jeans she was wearing. She was still finding it hard to take of her appearance and didn't care but now she felt a twinge of embarrassment. She looked a mess next to Serene.

Serene noticed her staring and seemed to read her thoughts. She reached out and put her hand on Laura's arm. "Listen, Laura; this is so weird - or maybe not so weird if you believe in destiny. Guess what I do? I'm a lifestyle coach and I specialize in depression and anxiety. I help people cure their depression and anxiety without medication."

Laura was stunned. It was weird; very weird that they should run into each other like this after all these years. She listened intently as Serene described how she had had helped dozens of people just like her overcome depression with lifestyle modifications without having to resort to prescription medication. She ran her business online, coaching and guiding her clients via one on one sessions via Skype and weekly group webinars.

"You might be wondering why I chose this field," she went on. "It's because I've been there. I suffered from severe depression in my early twenties. In fact, I was starting to have suicidal thoughts. I went to doctors, tried therapy, and was put on medication but it only messed me up more...until I went over the edge and tried to take my own life."

Laura started at her friend, dumbfounded. This gorgeous, articulate, sell-assured woman was saying that she had experienced what Laura was going through now! Serene explained how she had finally decided to fight back on her own terms and regain control of her life without medication. Through a process of trial and error, she devised an all-natural lifestyle routine that gradually pulled her out of depression and cured her for good. She had dedicated her life to helping others do the same.

"So you see," Serene concluded, "I've been there. I've been through hell and back so I know what it's like. And I guess you might say I'm living proof that anyone can overcome depression." Living proof! That was the understatement of the millennium. This beautiful, captivating woman with her bright eyes and calm wisdom was more than living proof! She was a living miracle.

"Look, Laura, this is not a sales pitch or anything. I have more clients than I can handle. But I' would love to help you if you will let me." It was a tempting offer but Laura was hesitant, her mind racing…was it worth the risk? She was getting better on the drugs already. Would it be wise to stop mid-track? And what would Alex say? He would be dubious to say the least. In fact, he'd probably insist that she continue with her doctor…Frankly, she herself was skeptical. She knew that depression medications worked directly on the brain chemicals which were causing illness. How could "lifestyle modifications" alter brain chemicals?

Gathering her thoughts, she thanked Serene for her offer but said she prefer to remain with her doctor for the time being as she was making progress. Serene did not seem to take it personally. In fact, she seemed to understand her thought process. "Just remember, I'm here if you ever do decide to try something different." They exchanged numbers, promised to meet up again soon. Serene left to finish her shopping and Laura headed home to prepare her husband's birthday dinner.

Chapter 3 – Friend to the Rescue

A month later, Laura called Serena weeping hysterically, begged for her help. She had made the bitter realization that drugs would not be enough to help her. Following that initial surge of improvement, things had started to go downhill.

She knew she was plunging into a downward spiral, she knew the drugs were making her worse but she kept telling herself that the medications needed time to work and that the doctor knew best. Her doctor seemed unconcerned. "These drugs do have some side effects," he had said, "but they are rarely serious and the end goal is what matters."

But she had always trusted her gut instinct and she just knew that the medications were making things worse. She had started binge eating and had gained 6 pounds. She felt bloated and ugly which only added to her depression. She was having mood swings where she would lash out at colleagues or at Alex for no good reasons. She wasn't sleeping well and would often toss or turn all night, shaking and sweating. But that was nothing compared to the black, gaping nothingness she felt inside. The terrifying chasm of numbness and despair was growing wider and wider, threatening to swallow her up g from the inside out and she would disappear forever as if sucked into a black hole. She stopped caring about anything; her looks, her friends, her job…and Alex. What was the point? There was no point to anything.

She took a month's leave from work and lay in bed all day, staring at the ceiling in between bouts of fitful sleep, only forcing herself to get up before Alex came home from work. She ignored his worried looks. She turned down her mother's invitation to go stay with her for a while. She didn't answer calls from friends. With each day the chasm grew bigger and deeper.

Until one morning she found herself staring at the three bottles of prescription pills lined up on her dresser. It would be so easy to just swallow the whole lot, one bottle after the other. Would she feel any pain or would she drift peacefully off?? What if Alex came home in time to rush her to the emergency room? Would a high building be better? Probably; it would be instant and guaranteed. What about a passing truck? No, too messy and she might live.

And as she sat there thinking of the easiest way to kill herself, it suddenly hit her what she was doing…she was planning how to end her life.

She ran to her phone to call her doctor but for some strange reason, she remembered Serene and called her instead. Within an hour, Serene was at her door.

They spent the afternoon talking. Laura poured out her feelings to her old friend who listened with tears in her eyes. What Laura was telling her was so similar to her own downward spiral that she became even more convinced that fate had indeed brought them together.

Serene promised that everything would be all right and that she would put her on a program of recovery right away. They waited for Alex to come home as he had a key role to play in Laura's battle. Finally, they heard his car in the driveway.

Brief introductions were made, and Laura told Alex what had been happening to her. She had seemed quite and detached lately and he had been thinking of suggesting she see another doctor. But he had never imagined he had come so close to losing his wife. Next, Serene explained who she was, what she had come to do and how crucial Alex's role would be in helping and supporting his wife. She said they needed to start right away. After getting over his initial shock, Alex picked up his phone and ordered pizza. "We'll talk over dinner," he said.

Chapter 4 – Starting The Five Pillars

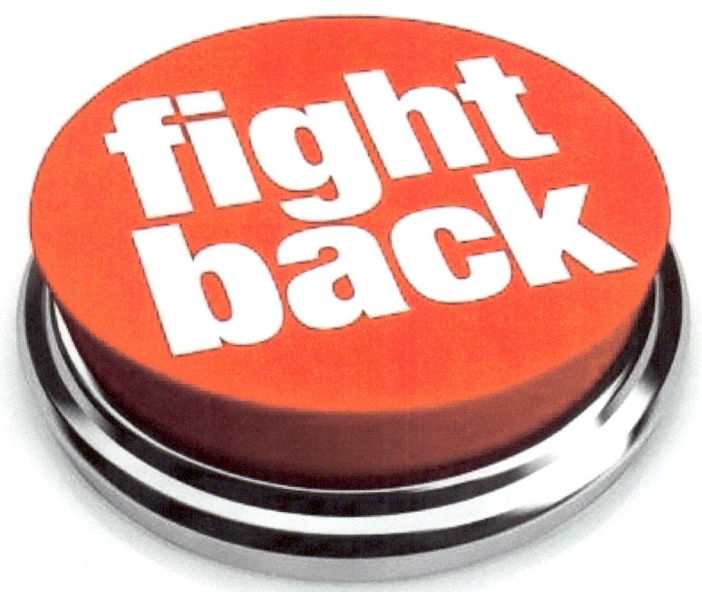

That same evening Serene outlined her unique program for combating depression, which included the same methods she herself had used to overcome her depression. She had developed and tweaked it over the years, making it easily adaptable to the circumstances of each individual client.

But first there was one thing Laura had to do – stop taking prescription medications immediately. "It's the best way to get off them once and for all," Serene explained, reassuring Laura that there would be no harm in this with the drugs she was taking. She would have some withdrawal symptoms for a week or so, but nothing more serious.

Laura cast a worried glance at Alex who apparently had the same thought. "Withdrawal symptoms? That sounds scary."

"That's right," Serene replied. "Laura has probably become addicted to the drugs. Going cold turkey is really the best option for getting those poisons out of her system." She assured them that the lifestyle changes Laura would make would kick in almost immediately to affect the brain chemicals in exactly the same way as the drugs - but without any of the harmful side effects she was feeling. "Remember," she said, "I've been there. Drugs are a waste of time and money unless you *really* need them, and I don't believe Laura does."

Alex still looked a bit skeptical. "If it's that simple then why are so many people taking these medications – and why are doctors prescribing them instead of a program like yours?"

Serene nodded in understanding. "Because we've become conditioned to believe that medicines are more potent and effective because they are based in 'scientific research and that our doctor knows best. But guess what? It's our ancestors who knew best way before medicines were invented. They looked to nature for safe and healthy options, and from personal experience I have come to trust and depend on natural alternatives."

Serene was not only speaking from personal experience. She had spent years researching and studying these methods that had worked for her and was able to confirm with clinical data and research findings that they were effective in all but very severe cases of depression and anxiety. In other words, her own success story convinces her even more.

Through that special eye language that married couples have, Laura communicated to Alex that she was convinced and ready to give it a try.

Serene's program was based on five pillars or steps that would be implemented one after the other over a series of weeks or months, depending on how quickly Laura was able to adapt to them. Laura could start immediately with the first and second pillars, which were essentially the foundation on which the other three pillars would be based. This foundation would help keep Laura on track and ensure that the results she achieved were long-lasting.

First, Laura and Alex needed to create a schedule of small daily tasks that Laura must stick to and accomplish. It is imperative that this schedule be established and adhered to, as a daily routine was proven to keep depressed persons focused, active and motivated. More tasks would be added to this schedule gradually. Serene gave the couple fifteen minutes to plan this schedule together and record it on Laura's laptop. They decided that Laura's main tasks for the coming week would be fixing breakfast, watering their houseplants at around noon, taking a short walk around the block later in the day and washing up after dinner. Alex volunteered to do the cooking or bring home takeout. This schedule would be expanded gradually as Laura made progress.

Now it was time for Pillar 1, which depended solely on Laura herself: deciding to fight back. She must make the commitment to fight against her depression and regain control of her life. Without a sincere and honest commitment on Laura's part, the program would fail. Serene looked Laura full in the eyes and her voice was soft but firm. "Swallowing a bunch of pills is so easy, isn't it? That's why medication doesn't work. People think it will miraculously cure with no effort on their part. Unless you make the decision to actively fight back, the cycles of depression will continue. This is going to take every ounce of your strength and willpower. There will be days when you will just want to give in. It's going to be an uphill struggle all the way. So Laura, You have to make a commitment here and now, to me, and Alex that you will fight back with all you've got."

Laura didn't hesitate for a heartbeat. She wanted nothing more than to get her old self back and be done with this nightmare. Looking at Serene and knowing that she had overcome the same ordeal, and everything she had just told them, had convinced Laura that this program may be just what she needed.

"I'm one hundred percent committed to this. I want to regain control of life more than anything. I promise I won't let you - or myself – down."

Serene nodded and turned to Alex. "This will be a tough time for you too, Alex. Just remember that your role is to support, encourage and be there for Laura but never force or pressure her. The key to Laura's recovery is that she must be willing to fight this battle of her own free will" Alex replied that he understood and would give Laura nothing but pure support.

Pillar 2 was to recruit and build a strong support group. Laura needed to create a support network of close friends and family who would be informed of Laura's condition and enlisted to help with support and encouragement. Again, Serene gave the couple a few minutes to make a list of these trusted people to call. The list included both of their families with whom they were very close, three of Laura's close friends and several of their neighbors.

A support network was crucial for empowering Laura, especially during the first months of the program. Serene also suggested online support groups where Laura could share her feelings and experiences with other people battling depression. She would email Laura with some links in case she ever felt the need for additional support.

With that, Serene stood up and after arranging to check in with Laura every other day, gave her a warm hug, wished her good luck and left. That night in bed, Alex held Laura in his arms, told her how much she meant to him and promised to do whatever it took to help her recover. "We're going to see this through together, Laura. Just know that you can always depend on me." Laura knew that he meant every word he said. Alex was a fighter; and for her sake and his she would become a fighter too.

The first week went well. Laura was able to stick to the daily schedule without too much trouble. Getting out for her short walk around the block was the hardest part but her neighbor Sally who was part of the support group, volunteered to accompany Laura. At exactly 3 p.m. each day, she would find Sally on her doorstep, her 8-month old son in his stroller and a bright smile on her face. Sally said the stroll was perfect for her as it made her son sleepy and ready for a long afternoon nap. They would stroll around the block for about 10 minutes and Laura had to admit that she always felt refreshed afterwards.

Luckily, she had no withdrawal symptoms after stopping her medication, the thing she and Alex had feared most. She supposed it was because she hadn't been taking the medications for that long.

The support she was getting was unbelievable. Her friends and family were literally competing with each other to help out. Rarely did Alex have to cook dinner; hardly did a day go by when a neighbor did not drop by with food. Alex's mother, who lived nearby, offered to help out with housecleaning, laundry and shopping whenever Laura wasn't feeling up to it. Laura's own parents who lived a distance away called almost daily to say they loved her. There were frequent text messages and emails from all these people as well, offering encouragement, prayers and support. She was overwhelmed by this outpouring of love and had to admit that it was motivating. Laura understood now why Serene had included this as part of the foundation. with so many people cheering her on, it would be hard for Laura to let them all down. On several days when she just couldn't bring herself to water the plants or was tempted to leave the dishes in the sink, she thought of Alex, her family and all the wonderful friends who were so eager to give of themselves and their time, and somehow found the strength to get the tasks done and stick to her schedule.

Chapter 5 – The Battle Continues

The following week she met Serene at a downtown café to start pillar three of her recovery program. As usual, Serene looked breathtaking in a light green a sweater and black skirt, her luxuriant streaked hair falling to her shoulders in gleaming waves. Laura was again conscious of her own drab appearance next to her friend. She was just too tired and listless to put any effort into her appearance and no longer really cared, but seeing Serene always sparked in her a slight twinge of envy. There was a time when she too looked as healthy and beautiful and took meticulous pains over her appearance. but that seemed ages ago. "I know I look a mess," she told her friend. I just can't find the energy to do much more than shower and brush my teeth."That's perfectly normal," Serene replied "and we're going to address that in this stage because that's part of the recovery process; because when you look good, you feel good."

Serene explained that over the following four to six weeks they would work on the physical side of her recovery and that this would be the hardest phase. "This phase will require some changes in your lifestyle which will be very daunting to you, although they're actually quite minor. In short, this is the diet and exercise phase."

"Oh my God," Laura said worriedly. I've never been to a gym in my life and I've never stuck to a diet for more than a week. Daunting is an understatement. Frankly I don't think I can do it." Serene smiled with amusement. "I hate formal exercise too but I still exercise almost every day. I walk, swim, cycle and I love hiking. And by diet I don't mean a formal diet, either. Let's talk about some of the physical activities you enjoy…"

Laura liked to swim and before her depression had enjoyed going for nature walks. They decided she would go to a local indoor pool one day a week, take a walk in the park on another day and on Saturdays, she would go hiking with Alex or walk to the farmers market. That came to three days a week. Serene advised that 15 to 20 minutes of each exercise would be enough and not to push herself. Laura relaxed a little on hearing this. Three days of light exercise seemed all right, especially since these were activities she enjoyed anyway.

Next, Serene handed Laura a piece of paper. "Your diet," she said. It wasn't a weekly or daily meal plan as Laura had expected but a simple a two-column list of foods to eat and foods to avoid. The foods to avoid included sugar, caffeine, alcohol and all types of processed foods. The foods to eat included brown rice and whole grain bread, turkey, eggs, leafy vegetable, herbal teas, fresh fruits (especially bananas) and a small bar of dark chocolate twice a week, among other things.

Laura was mildly surprised to see that many of the foods on the list were foods that she liked anyway. She was also surprised the chocolate was on the list, and Serene told her it was considered a "feel good" food for depressives, but not to overdo it. Laura sighed with relief. It would not be too much of an effort to eat these foods on a daily basis.

Serene explained that these specific foods helped the brain to release Serotonin, a chemical that promotes feelings of wellbeing and optimism. Exercise would increase her energy levels boost her drive and motivation as well as produce anti-depression chemicals in the brain. Together, both diet and exercise would help Laura's body physically combat her depression.

Next, Serene asked Laura to choose two more tasks to add to her daily schedule that would help Laura work on her appearance. They decided that Laura would give herself a deep facial cleaning one day a week and spend half an hour on her nails another day. Laura was to start phase two the very next day.

To Laura's dismay, she found herself beginning to struggle immediately. The next day, which had been scheduled for her swim, she simply could not muster up the will to do it. It would mean getting dressed, packing her swimsuit and towel, driving to the pool, changing then getting dressed again and coming home; it was just too huge of an effort for her. All she wanted was to curl up in bed and sleep for the rest of the morning. But Alex's mother had volunteered to accompany her and would be arriving any minute. Sure enough, the doorbell rang just minutes later. Alex's mother Carol stood smiling at the door. "Ready?" she asked. "I think this is a great idea. I could use the exercise" she added, slapping her thighs.

"Oh Carol, I'm so sorry for dragging you over like this but I'm really not up to it. Let's make it another time," Laura said. Carol wasn't going to give up so easily. "Now Laura, I know we're not supposed to pressure you but if you don't get your stuff and come with me right now, I'm going to kick your butt all the way down there. How's that for pressure?"

Laura found herself breaking into laughter. Carol's wry humor was one of the traits that endeared her to everybody. Carol patted her shoulder and her smile was warm and loving, "Come dear; the first step is always the hardest. You'll feel so much better afterwards, I promise."

Laura had to literally drag her feet upstairs to get dressed, drag her feet to the car and sat listlessly in the car during the short drive to the pool. But once in the warm water, swimming slowly back and forth, she did start to feel better. In fact, it was a full hour before she felt that she wanted to leave. Once back home, rather than dropping into bed as she had expected, she found herself pottering around the house, tidying up and putting a load of laundry in the machine. Carol had been right. She did feel better.

And so the cycles went. Each time her exercise day came around, she had to struggle so hard to get out of the house that her muscles literally ached. But once she was outdoor and moving around, she had to admit that she did start to feel better. The one day that she missed was her Saturday walk with Alex, when she just could not get out of bed. The look of disappointment and worry on his face was what made her force herself to get up the next time.

Those four weeks were the toughest in her life - emotionally and physically, but Serene seemed pleased and said she was doing very well. Laura could only trust her because she herself wasn't sure. Yes, there had been a lot of ups but there had equally been a lot if downs; but on the whole, she did feel better. The listlessness was still there but the periods of total desolation had become less frequent.

Thankfully, the diet part of this phase was a breeze. Both Alex and Laura were generally healthy eaters and had no trouble incorporating the prescribed foods into their diet. Saturday's walk to the local farmers market gave them the added bonus of stocking up on fresh fruits and vegetables for the week – as well as fresh honey, which Laura was using as a sweetener. By the third week, Laura noticed that she had lost a bit of her extra weight, which brought her a rare moment of pure joy.

Then one day during the fifth week, something amazing happened. Without realizing what she was doing, Laura jumped out of bed and found herself in the kitchen packing a light brunch for her hike with Alex that day. Slicing tomatoes, she suddenly froze with the knife mid-air as she realized what had happened – she was actually looking forward to the hike in the hills! She was actually preparing for it!

On Alternate Sundays, they had been driving to the outskirts of town and the surrounding hills, a beautiful nature area popular with hikers.

They would park the car, choose one of the trails leading up to the hills then walk back and drive home. It was these walks that Laura enjoyed the most. At first she could only walk for 10 or so minutes before turning back but lately they had been spending more and more time enjoying the wild beauty of the area. But soon winter would be here and that would have to wait for spring to resume their hikes.

And now, here she was making brunch for them to enjoy in their walk so that would not have to turn back home early. How and when did this happen? She didn't know but that moment was an eye-opener for her. She had been slowly improving. She had come a long way and she was more resolved than ever to win.

She ran – actually ran upstairs and shook Alex, who was still asleep. "Wake up, sleepyhead," she said in her old, cheerful voice. "It's time for our walk!" Alex groaned then realizing what she had said, sat bolt upright in bed, his eyes wide open with surprise. Laura laughed at him and ran back downstairs.

Chapter 6 – Harnessing The power from Within

Six weeks later, Laura began implementing the fourth pillar of the recovery program, which was the inner or spiritual aspect of her recovery. She was learning how to meditate – and she loved it! Ironically, she had never been a spiritual person and had always regarded yoga, meditation and other spiritual activities as somewhat bogus. They were a nice hobby if you enjoyed that type of thing but they weren't her cup of tea. She just didn't believe they were worth her time.

But Serene had explained that the physical changes Laura was making would not be enough on their own. Spiritual or inner wellbeing was essential for supplementing her recovery – it was inner strength and mental resolve that would ultimately help Laura win the battle, and these would be attained by focusing on the spiritual.

Serene introduced Laura to several options which included prayer, yoga and meditation. Laura chose meditation just because it seemed like the easiest, although she was still pretty skeptical about the whole thing.

Serene advised starting with five minutes of daily meditation sessions, and then building up to 15 minutes twice or three times a week. 15 minutes was the minimum for meditation to be effective. Laura would start practicing by just learning to focus on her breathing.

Serene gave her an audio CD of ocean waves breaking on the shore. All she had to do was inhale deeply while imagining the wave swelling and cresting then exhale as the wave washed onto the shore. She was to focus completely on inhaling and exhaling to the sound of the waves. The exercise was designed to teach the mind to focus inwardly on what the person was seeing and feeling.

The very first time Laura got ready to meditate, she felt a bit awkward and silly. She chose a time when she was alone at home, sat down in a comfortable chair with her legs stretched out like Serene had instructed and put on her headphones. She began inhaling and exhaling to the sound of the waves. About a minute later, she was completely immersed in the meditation, breathing deeply, feeling each breath as it left her lungs and each new breath entering her lungs. The sound of the ocean waves was relaxing and soothing. With her eyes closed, it was almost like she was sitting on a real shore in a beach chair and she could almost feel the wind in her face and the waves lapping at her feet...she became lost to everything else. She lost track of time, fully immersed in the beautiful tranquility she was feeling, until the recording ended. It had run for 15 minutes! So from the very first session, Laura went from being a total skeptic to becoming totally hooked on meditation. For the remainder of the week, she meditated for the full 15 minutes rather than the 5 minutes Serene had suggested.

Serene was very pleased but not surprised. "Most skeptics dismiss it until they've tried it," she said. "Personally, I don't think I could live without meditation."

Two weeks had passed and Laura was amazed at the transformation that was taking place in her. She was discovering an incredible, wondrous new world – not around her but inside of her! After the first week of practice, Serna had given her more recordings of more complex guided meditations or "visualizations" where she went on incredible spiritual journeys though lush valleys, mountains and forests teeming with magical waterfalls and clear streams, in which she would bathe and frolic. She would return from these magical inner journeys rejuvenated and refreshed, as well as awed by the beautiful places she had visited mentally.

She had tapped into an inner strength she never knew she had, and now she was learning to build it up. Under Serene's guidance she was also learning to practice mindfulness, training her brain to be aware of the here and now rather than live in the future or past. With all of this she was gaining an inner peace, calm and wisdom that she never knew she had.

Now she was meditating for an hour each day and looked forward to her sessions with eagerness. To those around Laura, the transformation was nothing short of miraculous. The spiritual peace she was developing seemed almost tangible to those around her. She would often find Alex looking at her with wonder, and bemusement

– and who could blame him? She herself was amazed at what was happening to her.

In addition to meditation, Serene was teaching her to practice mindfulness techniques in order to retrain her mind to always be in the present. This was another amazing discovery. By always being present she was rediscovering the world around her. She was learning to stop dwelling on the past, which was futile or worrying about the future, which was also futile. She was learning to keep her thoughts and senses open to what was happening in the moment, with total acceptance and calm. It was an amazing feeling, liberating and empowering because it made her feel strong enough to face anything.

Her walks and hikes became a combination of spiritual and physical. Her body benefitted from the exercise while her soul and senses took delight and pleasure in the sounds, sights and smells around her.

If anyone had told her a few months ago that that spiritual empowerment could help her cure depression, she would have laughed. Now she had experienced firsthand that this was possible.

She now understood how Serene's amazing program, like the pieces of a puzzle was meant to fit together to form a complete whole. This was journey that would continue throughout her life and she would be eternally grateful to Serene for helping her take the first steps.

The fifth pillar was by far the easiest one for Laura. Quite simply, it was staying off prescription drugs and avoiding alcohol. Serene did not need to explain how these two things would create havoc with her brain chemistry and slow down her recovery – or even stop it altogether. Quite simply, Laura had no intention of ever going back to prescription drugs, and not drinking was a small price to pay for the progress she had made. She gradually got into the habit of having plain water or lemonade with her meals instead of her usual glass of wine. She was never tempted to drink – all she had to do was remember the downward spiral she had been on only a few months before and she would simply realize that she never wanted to feel that way again.

Chapter 7 – Beginning a New Life

It was a sunny May afternoon as Laura got dressed for her weekly session with Serene at the usual downtown café. Actually, they planned to mix business with pleasure, and after their session they were going shopping for summer clothes, after which they were going to meet their husbands for dinner. To the delight of both women, Alex and Laura's husband Steve had become good buddies and spent most of their free times together.

Laura grabbed her handbag and took a last look at herself in the mirror. Her sleeveless peach-colored dress showed off her slim arms, lightly tanned by the summer sun. Her auburn hair was soft and shiny and the new shorter haircut framed her face perfectly. Her skin glowed with health thanks to her diet and exercise routine, and her eyes shine with the inner calm and tranquility she had found in meditation... She was beautiful. She felt beautiful, inside and out.

She intentionally arrived early, parking four blocks away from the café so that she could walk. Getting as much exercise as she could now came naturally to her and she no longer had to force herself to do it. She had recently bought a step tracker and wanted to get in as many steps as possible; she had challenged herself to get in a couple thousand steps than she had done the previous week.

Walking down the street, she found herself recalling her journey to recovery. Eight months had passed since that desperate phone call to Serene. Not only had she regained control of her life but she had become stronger, healthier and resolved never to fall into depression again. She would put the bad memories behind her; those early bleak days, the painful struggle for recovery, the tears and the hopelessness. Life was wonderful and she wanted to live it with every cell in her body. She knew that she had changed for good.

Serene was waiting for her at the cafe and when she saw her walk in, she beamed. "You look lovely! All dressed up for our last session, I see."

"Our last session? You didn't mention anything about that, Serene."

"Look at you," Serene replied. "What do you need me for? You're doing great! You don't need any more hand-holding. Now let's go shopping!"

On a personal level, Laura and Serene had revived their old friendship but now it was deeper and more intimate; it was the closeness of two mature women with a shared experience of a painful struggle.

Laura was absolutely convinced that destiny had played a role in reuniting them. She could not have recovered without her friend's selfless help, nor could anyone else have convinced her that it was possible to conquer depression with a simple, all-natural routine. As they left the café, Laura impulsively embraced her friend and whispered, "Thank you!" Serene returned the hug warmly and when she pulled away Laura saw that there were tears in her eyes.

They spent the next few hours happily shopping and sharing fashion advice. Before they knew it, it was time to meet their husbands at a nearby restaurant. When they walked into the restaurant laden with shopping bags, Laura noticed several men turn to look at them with admiration. She knew the glances were directed at her as well as her friend. She no longer felt ashamed of looking dowdy next to Serene. She knew she was just as confident, elegant and beautiful as Serene. She caught Alex's admiring glance across the room as well, and smiled. Admiring glances from other men were nice but knowing her husband thought she was beautiful was all she really cared about.

During dinner, Laura looked at the three people who meant so much to her, her heart swelling with love. Next to her was her beloved, wonderful husband who had been so patient and loving every step of the way. She knew that her ordeal had been a true test of his love for her and he had come through with flying colors. Across the table was Serene's husband Steve, the newest addition to their life. She knew how much he had supported and encouraged Alex when he was sick with worry over her. And next to Steve, her beautiful and loyal friend who had put all of this into motion. She knew that she was blessed to have these people in her life.

She looked at Alex and nodded; it was time. Alex cleared his throat dramatically.

"Guys, we've brought you here under false pretenses. I said that this was my treat but Steve, you have no choice but to foot the bill after you hear our announcement."

"Nothing short of you declaring bankruptcy will make me reach for my wallet," Steve shot back. "Laura's shopping bags suggest otherwise. So what's this amazing piece of news?"After a long moment of silence, Alex and Laura said together, "We're pregnant!"

Total chaos ensured. Serene started clapping wildly and knocked over her water glass. Steve reached out to slap Alex on the back, knocking over his water glass. Alex sat back and surveyed the scene with amusement and Laura burst out laughing. After the burst of excitement was over, Serene voiced what Laura was hoping to hear.

"I'm so happy for you guys. Knowing how responsible you both are only confirms that Laura has fully recovered. I know you would never have made this decision unless you felt you were ready for it. Congratulations."

Laura's happiness was complete. In fact, she wondered if she deserved so much happiness. Her spiritual awakening had triggered something inside her and she had explored the new feeling. She realized that more than anything else in the word, she wanted to be a mother. She knew, she was absolutely certain that she was ready just as she knew that Alex would be a wonderful father.

She had long thought about her purpose in life. She realized that it was not career, travel, material possessions that would fulfill her. Her fulfillment was in bringing a new life into this world, and to accompany her son or daughter on the beautiful journey that was life.

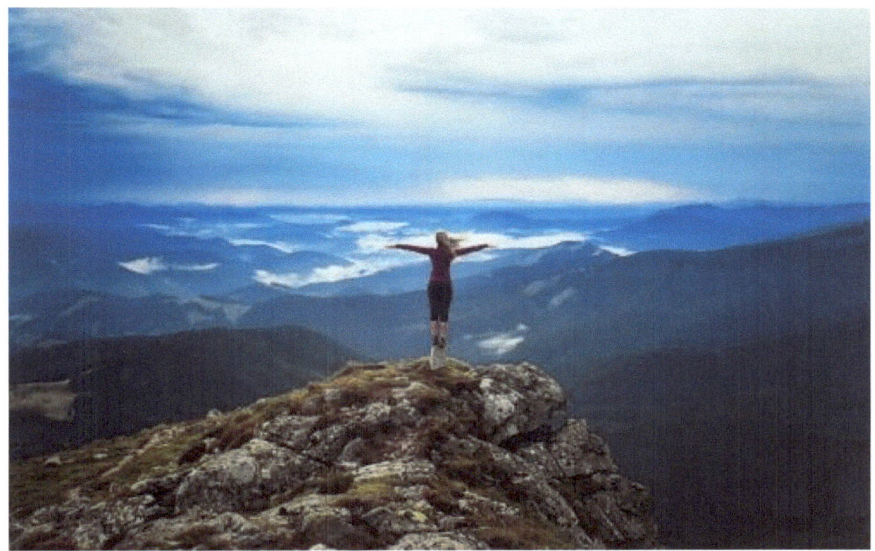

Epilogue

I hope you have enjoyed the story.

This book is meant as a companion book to my other book - Overpowering Depression and Anxiety : The Drug Free and Sustainable Way.

In that book, I outlined a battle plan for coordinated attack and fighting back on depression, and to make sure we win the battle in a sustainable way so that they do not come back to haunt us again. I introduced the 5 pillars strategy that are essential in this battle plan. It is meant to described clearly a strategy which you can use to defeat depression in a sustainable way.

However, some readers have commented that while the book is an easy and good read to make them understand the concepts, it does not show them or fully convince them that it can be done. They prefer stories that show more clearly how people actually apply these concepts.

Thus, the idea for this book was born. It is hoped that through an example of Laura's journey out of depression, readers can relate better to the concept introduced in the previous book. If you started from just reading the story in this book, but would like to understand the concepts behind this book better, then I also encourage you to pick up the earlier book, and compare the concepts in that book with this story.

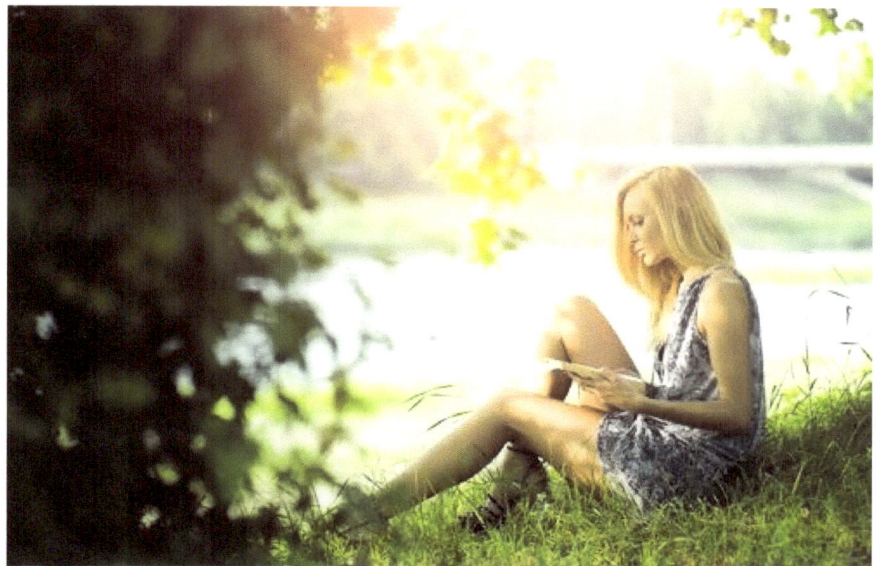

Yours Sincerely.

Serene Genie

www.ingramcontent.com/pod-product-compliance
Lightning Source LLC
Chambersburg PA
CBHW050845290526
45792CB00002B/529